LOSE WEIGHT AND KEEP IT OFF FOREVER

Tips and Tricks on Losing Weight and Winning a Lasting Healthy and Happy Lifestyle

PINK WOOL

Contents

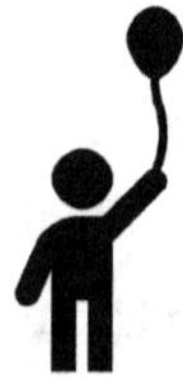

Chapter One

From Childhood to a Mind-Blowing Journey

A Child Holding on Strongly in the Wind

In the strong winter winds between blocks of flats, I clung to fences as a tiny, skinny girl, walking on my way to the tramway that took me to school. Little did I know that winds of change awaited me in adulthood, shaping my lifestyle and, ultimately, my weight.

Turning Points: Becoming a Wife and a Parent

Fast forward, many years later, moving in with my husband marked the beginning of subtle changes in our lifestyle, and the gradual accumulation of extra weight became noticeable in less than a year. Mostly sedentary lifestyle and great quantities of amazing food plus scrumptious desserts. However, an even bigger shift happened after I gave birth to my son and my first child.

Packing on a bit over 10 kilograms during pregnancy kicked off a phase of hectic parenting, where careful and mindful eating, active lifestyle and workouts took a backseat. Does it sound familiar?

A Pause and a Restart: The Birth of Transformation

Fast forward again - nearly six years, and my second baby entered the scene of our lives. With a big desire, but no practical, proven formula to shed the extra weight, I found myself back at square one, if not worse. Unaware of the journey ahead, I embarked on a new chapter of my life.

My Hunt for Weight-Loss Answers

For many years, I sought explanations about my stubborn weight, complained about the lack of time and motivation, blamed my contraceptive pills, explored, and tried various diets, and overanalyzed the reasons behind my weight struggles. Mummy tummy and untoned arms haunted me. Frustration set in, exacerbated by the temporary successes of various diets and exercise phases. If you're reading this book, I guess you know what I'm talking about. It's a common narrative we've all experienced.

The Zumba Interlude

Zumba, a beacon of hope, entered my life at some point as I was watching TV. A couple of DVDs, I bought after watching that TV program, and after that, a few local live classes added rhythm to my workouts, introducing joy into my fitness routine at home and at a local venue with like-minded people. And new hope. Yet, the tricky weight-loss solution remained hidden until the day when I stumbled upon a serendipitous Facebook post.

A Life-Changing App: Noom

A Facebook ad introduced me to Noom, an app promising a lifestyle change backed by science. I completed a survey and I received a plan tailored to my weight goal and my existing lifestyle. Skepticism shifted to hope (again!) and a more palpable promising future during the free trial. The first two weeks brought visible weight loss and showed me the app's scientific foundation and very easy-to-understand steps and lessons, including quick, useful meal tracking.

Please note that I didn't write this book to pitch Noom or convince anyone to try it unless you genuinely believe it aligns with your needs. Moreover, there might be other thousands of apps or programs like that out there. It's more than this in this book, it's about how a little but significant success boosted my confidence and brought a holistic change to my whole life, health, and relationships.

Chapter Two

Setting Goals and Breaking Limits

My initial goal of losing 5 kilograms in three months was surpassed within a month, fuelling a newfound determination to aim higher. Noom's holistic approach, featuring coach and peer support, nutritional insights, and exercise and food tracking, suited and captivated me. I was so motivated, fascinated and inspired. I talked non-stop about it. Finally, I started believing it was possible to lose weight - with all my heart, body and soul.

What I think made my trial a success was setting a SMART goal. Just in case you haven't heard of or you need a little refresher on what these SMART goals are, why and how they work, here is a brief breakdown.

Setting SMART goals is a framework that helps individuals and organizations define clear objectives and increase the likelihood of achieving them. SMART is an acronym that stands for Specific, Measurable, Achievable, Relevant, and Time-bound. Here's how to set SMART goals and why they work:

- **Specific (S):**

Define your goal with clarity and precision. Be clear about what you want to achieve.

Ask yourself: What exactly do I want to accomplish? Why is it important? Who is involved? Where will it happen? What resources or limits are involved?

- **Measurable (M):**

Establish concrete criteria for measuring progress toward the attainment of each goal.

Ask yourself: How will I know when the goal is accomplished? What metrics will I use to measure progress?

- **Achievable (A):**

Ensure that the goal is realistic and attainable given the resources, time, and circumstances.

Ask yourself: Can I realistically achieve this goal? Do I have the necessary support, skills and resources?

- **Relevant (R):**

Make sure that the goal matters and aligns with your broader objectives or values.

Ask yourself: Is this goal worthwhile and aligned with my broader objectives? Is it the right time to pursue this goal?

- **Time-bound (T):**

Set a specific time frame for achieving the goal to create a sense of urgency.

Ask yourself: By when do I want to achieve this goal? What can I do today, this week, and this month to move toward my goal?

Why SMART Goals Work

Clarity:
SMART goals provide a clear and concise definition of what needs to be achieved. This clarity helps in understanding the desired outcome.

Focus:
The specificity of SMART goals helps individuals and teams to stay focused on what needs to be done, reducing distractions and irrelevant activities.

Motivation:
SMART goals can be motivating because they are realistic and achievable. People are more likely to stay committed to goals they believe they can reach.

Measurement and Evaluation:
The measurable aspect of SMART goals allows for objective assessment. Progress can be tracked and adjustments made as needed.

Accountability:
The time-bound nature of SMART goals creates a sense of urgency and accountability. It helps in avoiding procrastination and encourages timely action.

Alignment:
SMART goals are designed to be aligned with broader objectives, ensuring that individual or team efforts contribute to larger personal or organizational goals.

By incorporating these principles, SMART goals provide a structured and effective way to plan, execute, and evaluate progress towards desired outcomes, in our case, weight loss.

Another great trick I learned along the way from my weight loss and fitness journeys: Break your goal down into even smaller goals, more achievable, faster. You can determine how and where to start by thinking: can I lose 2.5 kg in one month or walk 30 min a day? If you have any doubts, then reduce the goal: can I lose 2 kg in one month and walk 20 min a day? Do this until you feel comfortable with your goal and start from there. Then, a magic thing will happen when you achieve your smaller goal! You will have proof that you can achieve something meaningful. You will start thinking, "I lost those 2 kgs in one month, I can do it again this month, it's doable!". This is how you build your self-confidence which is so important during these health journeys and any project in your life. Don't forget to celebrate your achievement!

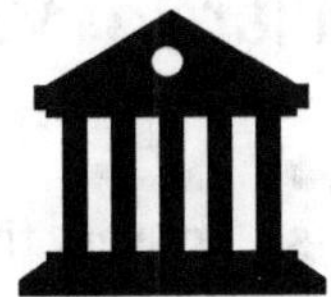

Chapter Three

The Pillars of Wellness

Everything made sense to me finally. All my questions were answered. Noom's emphasis on four pillars—nutrition, fitness, sleep, and stress management—resonated deeply with me and my lifestyle. Noom's Chief of Psychology, Andreas Michaelides, Ph.D., highlighted the importance of a full mind-body approach to optimal health: "At Noom, we believe that achieving optimal 'health' requires tending to four key pillars: **nutrition, fitness, sleep, and stress management**, which is why we promote a full mind-body approach within our curriculum". A couple of years later, after reading tons of books and listening to an infinite list of podcasts on health and happiness, I learned that there is another pillar that we all should add to our wellbeing foundation: **nurturing our relationships.** What contributes to a life marked by happiness, fulfillment, and goodness? The directors of the Harvard Study of Adult Development, the most extensive scientific inquiry into happiness, suggest that the answer to this question may be more accessible than commonly thought.

The key to a meaningful and fulfilling life? Relationships emerge as the unexpectedly simple yet powerful answer. The Harvard Study of Adult Development finds that the strength of our connections with others significantly influences our likelihood of leading a joyful, gratifying, and overall healthier life. In fact, this study indicates that the strength of our interpersonal bonds can serve as a reliable predictor of both our physical and cognitive wellbeing throughout our life journey. I highly recommend you read "The Good Life: Lessons from the World's Longest

Scientific Study of Happiness" by Robert Waldinger, Marc Schulz.

A Priceless Investment in My Wellbeing

I must admit that I wasn't very happy to spend any amount of money on weight loss programs. And I also firmly believed in finding ways to achieve my goals without significant expenditure or even zero costs. The fact that I could explore the app for free during the initial week or two was a game-changer. Additionally, I procrastinated on subscribing until the last possible day, and fortunately, I secured a discount for the three-month plan.

While the cost exceeded what I'd typically spend on personal experiences and gifts, my belief and strong hope in the program's effectiveness led me to rationalize the expense. Breaking it down over three months made the monthly cost more manageable in my mind. Interestingly and funnily enough, during my Noom journey, I referred numerous family members and friends to join and start their own journeys, essentially offsetting my initial subscription cost with the value of the Amazon vouchers I earned.

I'll always remember the sense of accomplishment as I collected those vouchers in my Amazon account. They allowed me to purchase a fantastic pair of Puma running shoes that became a symbol of pride and achievement. These shoes not only stood as a tangible reward but also added an extra layer of motivation and inspiration to my entire journey as I used them for my running.

The Power of Mindful Eating

What drew me towards this fresh approach to weight loss was the assurance that I could still indulge in my favorite foods – a rare feature in most diets. The rationale behind it was straightforward: resisting certain foods often triggers intensified cravings, leading to overeating beyond genuine satisfaction. The journey also exposed me to new concepts and experiences like **mindful eating**, a revelation that went beyond calorie counting. Balancing nutrition, understanding Ghrelin (the hunger hormone that I heard of for the first time during that period of my life), and savoring every bite became important aspects of my wellbeing evolution.

A Holistic Approach

In the past few years, particularly since embarking on my journey to a healthier lifestyle, I've come to realize that there's no one-size-fits-all solution to losing weight. What worked for me succeeded because I committed to making it work, staying determined to reach my goals. I adhered to the new rules in nutrition with discipline, remained open to learning about the impact of food on my weight and wellbeing, and implemented small but important changes across all aspects of my life. Despite facing a few challenges along the way, I trusted the process, sought answers, did my own research, and most importantly, I celebrated every small and significant achievement when it happened.

In a nutshell, the synergy of balanced nutrition, a calorie deficit, and regular exercise formed the heart of my weight loss. This powerful strategy not only shed excess weight but also nurtured a healthier and more resilient body. My journey, shared in this book, aims to inspire and motivate you too, proving that transformation is within reach for anyone on the path to better health.

Chapter Four

Breaking Down My Initial 90-Day Weight Loss Success

As essential as the app was to my success, I'm eager to walk you through how the whole process worked and the invaluable lessons I gained during those challenging but rewarding 90 days, a journey of self-discovery.

Balanced Nutrition: Beyond the Eye Roll

Let's start by talking about the importance of balanced nutrition and the crucial role of a calorie deficit in the weight loss process. Initially skeptical, I used to dismiss talks of calorie counting with an eye roll. What a waste of time, I used to think. You need to be really desperate to be doing this, I used to think. If I eat healthy food, it should be enough to lose weight, I used to think. Little did I know that balanced nutrition is fundamental for overall health and especially weight loss. Including a variety of nutrients in appropriate proportions and even smaller portions was what I needed to start looking into.

Caloric Intake Management: The Deficit Game

Understanding and managing caloric intake played a central role in my journey. The concept of a calorie deficit, achieved by consuming fewer calories than burned, became my weight loss friend. Monitoring and controlling my intake allowed me to tap into stored fat for energy, generating effective weight loss.

A Revelation: I Was Eating Too Much Healthy Food!

Discovering where I went wrong was enlightening. All this time, I thought I was eating healthy, but in reality, I was unknowingly overly consuming healthy food. Mindless snacking, like absentmindedly eating almonds while working on the computer, became an issue in my weight loss. It was through this journey that I discovered and embraced mindful eating – appreciating flavors, colors, and textures... and – more than everything - decent, acceptable amounts. Ok, ten almonds and put the container back in the drawer! Eat them slowly: look at them, even smell them, and bite small bits, chew properly. There you go!

Quality Matters: Not All Calories Are Equal

Not all calories are created equal, and focusing on their quality is paramount. Here is a classic example. A handful of grapes is not the same as a handful of raisins. Grapes, similar to watermelon, boast high water content, reducing their caloric density and enhancing satiety without significantly contributing to your daily calorie intake. This fullness discourages reaching out for snacks with higher caloric density, hindering progress toward your weight loss goals.

To demonstrate the impact of water content on calories, let's compare a serving of grapes with a serving of raisins. Grapes contain 85% water, with 1 cup totaling 62 calories. In contrast, raisins, with only 15% water content, pack 434 calories per cup. This stark 600% difference shows the importance of water content in managing caloric intake, as raisins lack the satiating effect provided by grapes.

So choosing to eat not only healthier but smarter and having nutrient-dense foods — rich in essential vitamins and minerals — became a cornerstone of my dietary approach. A well-rounded nutritional diet involving fruits, vegetables, lean proteins, and whole grains became key. Wow!

How I Earned My Sweet Rewards

Additionally, integrating regular physical activity into my routine amplified the impact of a calorie deficit. This is where exercise became my friend. Recognizing that if I craved a slice of cake or an ice-cream or chocolate or the list could go on and on, I needed to counterbalance it with a long walk, a good run, or a lively Zumba session <u>on the same day</u> became a game-changer. The key is immediacy — I did the exercise to burn the extra calories right then and there, not the next day or during the weekend. Two essential principles emerge: offset extra calorie intake with on-the-day physical exercise and consider it a reward earned. It may sound like a joke, but this approach encouraged my discipline.

Oh, by the way, did I mention? It turns out there's scientific backing to this. After exercising, hunger tends to diminish, making indulging in sweets less tempting. Many times, I didn't even want the sweets anymore. Give it a shot!

Anyway, beyond calorie burning, exercise contributes significantly to overall health by enhancing cardiovascular fitness, fortifying muscle strength, and promoting mental wellbeing. So it's up to you how you want to frame and re-frame this approach.

Exposing My Misconceptions

As I mentioned already, calorie counting wasn't my belief system before starting this journey. I dismissed the idea as a tedious waste of time, considering myself a genuine consumer of healthy foods. However, this program challenged my perception, demonstrating that every morsel and sip matters. Grappling with inconvenience, I committed to measuring, weighing, and calculating calories for each meal, even extending the hassle to my drink choices. Yes, I have to confess, it was a useful exercise. Ah, and I was so judgemental... Ok, lesson learned. I was surprised to find out that I needed to add even my drinks to my daily calorie count. My orange juice, it's so healthy! How does that make me gain weight? Well, a glass of orange juice has 110 calories...

Initially daunting, this practice soon became second nature. I even discovered that a glass of wine carries a caloric load similar to that of my glass of orange juice - a revelation that shattered my belief in the presumed healthiness of certain choices. Even my seemingly innocent habit of consuming milk turned into a lesson; its full-fat (whole milk) version significantly outpaced the low-fat alternative in calories, 155 calories versus 108 per 250 ml. It might not seem like a lot, but it all adds up, that's another lesson I learned.

Breaking Generational Food Customs

Intriguingly, our eating habits often stem from childhood customs. In my family, wasting food was taboo, a tradition driven by scarcity but also an appreciation for the effort made by my parents to buy and prepare food for us. The "clean your plate" mentality persisted until I eventually managed to make myself embrace the concept of leaving the table with an 80% full stomach—a difficult but liberating shift in perspective. More about this new concept, new to me, further in this book.

Meal Adjustments for Weight Loss

Gradually, meal by meal, I fine-tuned my approach, manipulating quantities, food types, and proportions to align with my weight loss objectives. Dairy, a calorie-heavy culprit, saw a great reduction, with an inclination toward low-fat options and smaller quantities. The entire meal preparation process transformed into a nutritional experiment, making sure I was not consuming too much of even the healthiest foods any longer. For instance, instead of using whole milk to make my porridge for breakfast, I started using low-fat milk, actually only half the usual quantity, and adding water on top. Honestly, the taste didn't change significantly, but the number of calories decreased quite a bit. Smart, right?

The Beauty of Meal Tracking

Calculating and weighing food became the most challenging yet indispensable aspects of my journey. Despite the initial challenges, consistent tracking proved satisfying. I noticed patterns of overeating or under-consumption of certain foods, offering invaluable insights for healthy adjustments. Discoveries ranged from excessive quantities of olive oil in my salad dressings, or on my roast vegetables to realizing how much veggies and fruits I could eat and still keep within my daily calorie allowance.

Are there calorie-free foods?

This question often lingers in the minds of many embarking on their weight loss journey. I was amongst these people. While the concept of "calorie-free" may sound like a dream for those striving to shed pounds, the reality is a bit more nuanced.

In the world of nutrition, no food is truly calorie-free. Even the most seemingly innocent choices have some caloric content. Disappointing, right? However, there are foods with such minimal calories that the energy expended in digesting them may surpass the calories they provide. These are often referred to as "negative-calorie" foods.

Common examples of negative-calorie foods include leafy greens like spinach and kale, celery, or zucchini and cucumbers, and certain fruits such as berries and grapefruit. These foods are rich in essential nutrients, fiber, and water, promoting a sense of fullness and aiding in digestion. Incorporating these into your diet can be a smart strategy for weight loss, as they offer a satisfying crunch without contributing significantly to your overall calorie intake. This sounds a bit more encouraging, right? It's actually awesome!

One more thing to keep in mind: it's crucial to approach the idea of negative-calorie foods with a balanced mentality. While they can be valuable additions to your diet, they should not be the sole focus of your nutrition plan. It happened to me though, so don't make the same mistake. Successful weight loss involves a holistic approach that considers not only the quantity, but also the quality and the variety of the calories consumed.

In the upcoming sections and chapters, we'll dig deeper into the science of nutrition and weight loss by exploring the role of macronutrients and micronutrients, and provide practical tips to help you make informed choices on your journey to a healthier, fitter you. Remember, the key lies not in eliminating calories entirely, but in understanding and managing them wisely.

Fuelling Properly: The Crucial Role of Macronutrients and Micronutrients in Your Weight Loss Journey

In the pursuit of a healthier and happier self, understanding the significance of macronutrients and micronutrients is very important. These nutritional building blocks form the foundation of your body's function, affecting not only your weight but also your overall wellbeing. Let's see what role they play in your weight loss journey and the creation of a lasting, healthy lifestyle.

Macronutrients

Macronutrients are the three main components of our regular diet that provide the energy necessary for daily activities. They include carbohydrates, proteins, and fats. Balancing these macronutrients is crucial for sustaining energy levels, promoting metabolism, and supporting muscle growth.

1. **Carbohydrates:** Often misconceived as the enemy in weight loss, carbohydrates are, in fact, a primary energy source. When you opt for complex carbohydrates such as whole grains, fruits, and vegetables you ensure a steady release of energy and promote satiety.

2. **Proteins**: Vital for muscle repair and growth, proteins play a pivotal role in weight loss. Lean protein sources like chicken, fish, legumes, and tofu can help you feel full longer, reducing the likelihood of overeating.

3. **Fats**: Healthy fats are essential for nutrient absorption, brain function, and hormone production. Include sources like avocados, nuts, seeds, and olive oil in your diet to support these vital functions while managing your weight effectively.

Micronutrients

While macronutrients provide energy, micronutrients are the vitamins and minerals that keep your body running smoothly. These micronutrients are important for various physiological processes, including metabolism, immune function, and bone health.

1. **Vitamins**: Essential for overall health, vitamins contribute to processes such as energy metabolism and immune system function. Incorporate a

diverse range of fruits, vegetables, and whole foods to ensure you receive a spectrum of vitamins.

2. **Minerals**: Minerals, like calcium, iron, and magnesium, are vital for bone health, oxygen transport, and muscle function. Include a variety of nutrient-dense foods such as dairy products, lean meats, and leafy greens to meet your mineral needs.

In your weight loss journey, recognizing the important role of both macronutrients and micronutrients is crucial for success. Strive for a balanced and varied diet, focusing on whole, nutrient-dense foods that provide the energy and essential elements your body needs to thrive. By understanding and embracing the power of these nutritional components, you pave the way for not only shedding unwanted weight but also fostering a sustainable and lasting healthy lifestyle.

Precision Nutrition or How to Tailor Your Plate for Weight Loss and Performance

Even if many of us are sports-orientated people, meaning we do sports, not only watch them on TV or go to see our favorite team playing at the local stadium, we still struggle with extra weight. This situation is quite frustrating and also tricky. This section is for those who want to know more about how to juggle between eating for weight loss and eating for sustainable energy which is required on a normal day but mainly on your training, race or game day. Because you want to or have already started your weight loss journey, you need to understand the dynamic relationship between macronutrients and your plate and how it becomes a key factor in achieving success. Whether you're enjoying a rest day, engaging in easy training, tackling moderate exercise, or preparing for a hard training session or even a race day, the proportions of protein, whole grains, and fruits and vegetables on your plate play a crucial role in fuelling your body, promoting weight loss, and optimizing performance.

Rest Day or Easy Training

On days when rest or light training takes center stage, it's important to focus on maintaining a balanced diet that supports recovery and nourishes your body without overloading it with excess calories. Emphasize lean protein sources like chicken, fish, or plant-based alternatives, complemented by a mix of whole grains such as quinoa or brown rice. Incorporate an array of colorful vegetables to provide essential vitamins and minerals, promoting overall wellbeing.

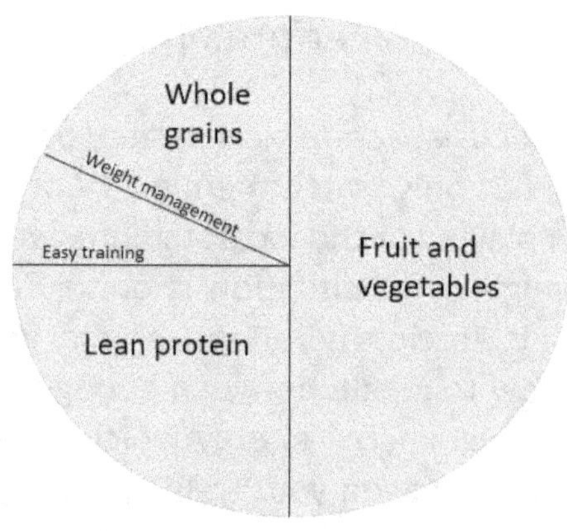

Moderate Training

When engaging in moderate training, your body requires a slightly elevated intake of energy to support increased activity levels. Adjust your plate to include a well-balanced combination of lean proteins, whole grains, and a variety of fruits and vegetables. This ensures a steady release of energy, aids muscle repair, and helps control hunger, ultimately contributing to effective weight management.

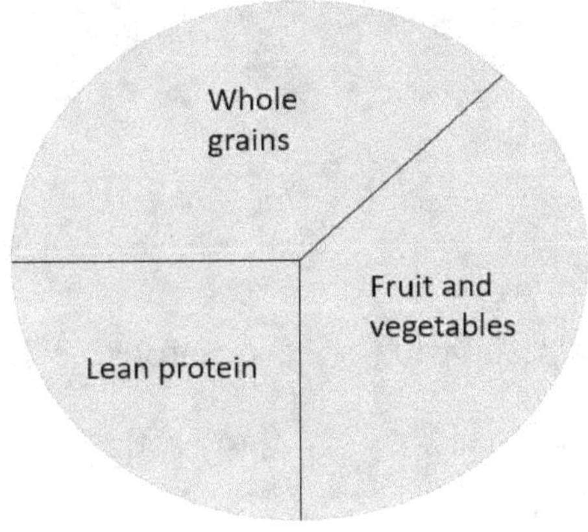

Hard Training or Race/Game Day

For intense training sessions or race/game days, fuelling your body with the right nutrients becomes crucial. Increase your carbohydrate intake with whole grains and fruits to provide readily available energy. Maintain an adequate amount of protein for muscle repair and include easily digestible fruits and vegetables to support hydration and micronutrient needs. Balancing these elements helps optimize performance and aids in recovery post-exercise.

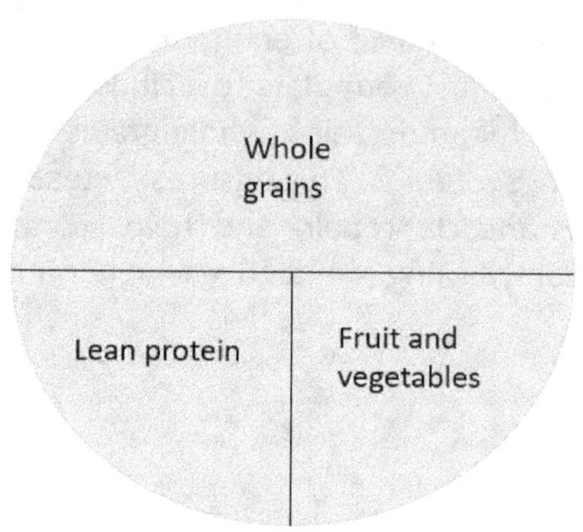

Whole grains: pasta, rice, potatoes, cereals, breads, legumes

Lean protein: chicken, beef, lamb, fish, eggs, low-fat diary, legumes, nuts, tofu

Vegetables and fruits: raw veggies, cooked veggies, veggie soup, fresh fruit

Weight Loss Emphasis

In the context of weight loss, portion control and mindful eating are very important. While adjusting macronutrient proportions based on activity levels, focus on maintaining a slight calorie deficit for effective weight loss. Prioritize lean proteins to preserve muscle mass, incorporate whole grains for sustained energy, and load up on fibrous fruits and vegetables to enhance satiety and nutrient intake.

Adapting your plate to reflect the demands of different training days is a powerful strategy for achieving both weight loss and performance goals. By understanding the nuanced requirements of your body during rest, easy training, moderate exercise, and intense workouts or game days, you can tailor your nutrition to support optimal health, enhance your fitness journey, and pave the way for lasting success in your weight loss undertaking.

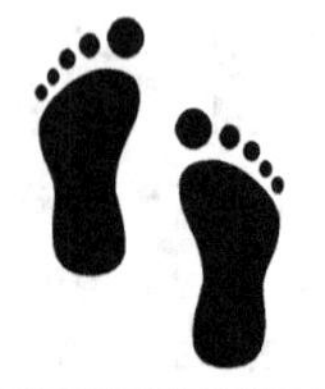

Chapter Five

Five Quick and Practical Tips for Success

When I decided to go on this revolutionary journey towards a healthier lifestyle, I would have wanted someone to show me what the most important steps to take were and why not, a few shortcuts. So here are a few lessons I learned that involve more than just nutritional insights, five quick and practical tips that served as my guiding lights. These strategies aren't complex; instead, they offer simplicity and effectiveness, making them seamlessly integrate into your daily routine.

1. **Combo Habit:** Blend necessary tasks or habits like exercise with enjoyable activities, such as calling a friend or listening to an audiobook when you go for a walk or even for a run. Take a Zumba class together with your friend.

2. **Low-Calorie Food Choices:** Put together a list of low-calorie fruits and vegetables, meats and dairy products and keep combining them to make salads or entire dishes.

3. **Hydration First:** Always drink a glass of water before meals to manage hunger.

4. **Simplicity in the Early Days:** Stick to straightforward, simple meals and recipes for the initial months so you can track them easily and spend less time preparing them. Or if you have no time at all to deal with this, you could even buy meals from the supermarket that have their

number of calories per serving written on the label. Make sure they are healthy.

5. **80% Full Rule:** Embrace "Hara hachi bu" — the Japanese practice of eating until 80% full, promoting mindful consumption. This is a real game-changer.

"Hara hachi bu" is a Japanese expression translating to "Eat until you're 80% full." Originating in Okinawa, this concept serves as a guide for individuals in managing their eating habits. Interestingly, those adhering to this practice in Okinawa experience notably low rates of heart disease, cancer, and stroke, contributing to a relatively long life expectancy in the region.

This multifaceted journey not only transformed my relationship with food and made me create for myself an active lifestyle, but also encouraged me to share these insights, hoping to inspire healthier paths for people like you.

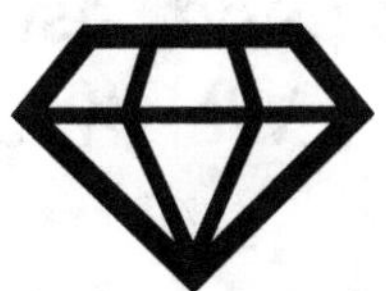

Chapter Six

Building Good and Lasting Habits: Key Practices for Weight Loss Success

Getting on a weight loss journey is not only a temporary change in your eating habits; it's a transformative process that requires a shift in lifestyle. One of the cornerstones of a successful weight loss journey lies in the formation of good habits.

Habits are powerful because they shape our daily routines and, over time, become ingrained in our behavior. When striving for weight loss, cultivating positive habits can make all the difference. Here's why:

Consistency is Key: Habits thrive on repetition. By consistently making healthier food choices and engaging in regular physical activity, you create a sustainable pattern that contributes to your overall wellbeing. Consistency builds momentum, making it easier to stick to your weight loss goals in the long run.

Automating Healthy Choices: Establishing good habits helps automate the decision-making process. When healthy behaviors become second nature, you're less likely to succumb to impulsive and potentially detrimental choices. Over time, the conscious effort required to make positive decisions diminishes as healthy habits become routine. Like brushing your teeth twice a day.

Stress Reduction: Any change can be challenging, and a weight loss journey often involves breaking free from old, less healthy patterns. Habits provide a sense of structure and predictability, reducing the stress associated with making constant decisions about what to eat or whether to exercise. When healthy choices become habitual, they become a natural part of your lifestyle, eliminating the mental strain of constant decision-making.

Long-Term Success: Weight loss is not only a destination; you will still need to look after yourself to keep your ideal weight so it's becoming a lifelong journey. Establishing good habits is crucial for maintaining your achievements over the long term. Crash diets and extreme workout routines might yield rapid results, but without sustainable habits, maintaining that progress becomes a difficult challenge.

In the chapters ahead, we'll explore practical strategies for cultivating positive habits, breaking free from detrimental ones, and creating a supportive environment that reinforces your commitment to a healthier you. Remember, building good habits is not just about reaching your ideal weight; it's about embracing a lifestyle that promotes lasting health and wellbeing.

In my weight loss journey, I established and maintained several habits that have been very helpful in achieving my goals and keeping my extra weight off. Here are the key practices I've learned about, I was happy with and incorporated into my daily routine:

1. **Daily Weigh-Ins:** Regularly using the scale to monitor my weight has provided invaluable insights into my progress, helping me stay accountable and adjust my approach as needed. When I had a party or a big dinner the night before, usually that was obvious in the number on the scale, so I made sure I was more careful with my

calorie intake that day. Most of the time though, this moment of the day is an opportunity for celebration: I lost a few grams or I maintained my weight! Happy time!

2. **Consistent Exercise Routine:** Incorporating daily exercise into my routine has not only contributed to calorie burning, but has also enhanced my overall wellbeing and my social life. Whether attending energizing Zumba classes with friends, taking leisurely walks filled with conversations or introspections, or connecting with overseas friends over the phone during a stroll, these moments have significantly contributed to my overall happiness and success in shedding extra weight.

3. **Stay Hydrated**: Prioritizing hydration by drinking lots of water and herbal tea has not only supported my metabolism, but has also helped curb unnecessary snacking by keeping me feeling full and satisfied. Sometimes when we think we are hungry, we are actually thirsty, so it's always a good idea to drink a glass of water or a cup of our favorite herbal or green tea before we reach for a snack.

4. **Mindful Alcohol Consumption**: I generally like a good dessert and I used to also have a glass of wine at dinner time. Knowing my sweet tooth, I made a conscious decision to reduce my alcohol intake instead, meaning no alcohol at all most days, to reduce calorie consumption. I have always

preferred an ice cream or a slice of cake over a glass of wine, so I didn't feel I missed out on much.

5. **Smart Chocolate Choices:** Exploring all the dark chocolate options on the market instead of consuming milk or white chocolate, which I found too sweet anyway, has allowed me to indulge my sweet cravings with a healthier alternative, one that is lower in sugar and higher in antioxidants. Plus, I don't know anyone who can eat lots of dark chocolate, I usually stop at square number two or three, ok four if the chocolate is that good. It's so rich and satisfying at the same time.

6. **Whole Grain Swaps:** Eating wholemeal pasta, wholemeal bread, and brown rice instead of their white counterparts has not only increased the nutritional value of my meals, but also contributed to a more stable and sustained energy release. They usually have the same amount of calories, can you believe it, but their nutritional value is much higher. I realize they might not be everyone's cup of tea, but it's an acquired taste. You will get used to the texture and taste and combined with vegetables or healthy sauces, the wholemeal pasta and brown rice are not bad at all.

7. **Emphasis on Salad:** Prioritizing healthy salads over heavier side dishes like rice or potatoes when accompanying my meat helps control calorie intake while ensuring a diverse range of nutrients in my

meals. I'm talking about simple salads, with vinaigrette dressing and not the ones loaded with mayonnaise or cheese-based dressings. So if you go to a restaurant and you order a salad, don't forget to ask the waiter to bring the dressing separately.

8. **Lean Protein Choices:** Whenever possible, I choose lean meats or fish as my protein sources. This not only supports muscle maintenance, but also helps control overall calorie intake. If you cannot give up the fatty meat or skin-on chicken breast or chicken wings straight away, try to eat only half of the amount you used to and for the other half introduce lean meat.

9. **Sugar-Free Dessert Choices:** Opting for desserts with no added sugar or just fruit, when available, allows me to satisfy my sweet tooth without compromising my effort to reduce unnecessary sugars in my diet.

These habits have collectively formed the foundation of my weight loss success, providing a holistic and sustainable approach to achieving and maintaining a healthier lifestyle. By incorporating these practices into my daily life, I've not only shed excess weight in a very short time, but also cultivated habits that contribute to my overall wellbeing even now, three years after that moment. I hope they are established for life and they help you too.

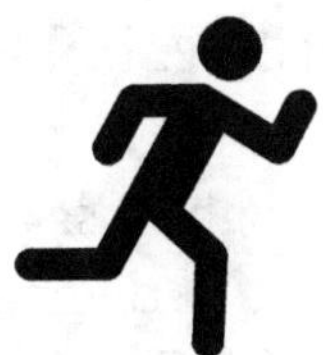

Chapter Seven

My Exercise Is Not Boring

In the pursuit of my weight loss goal, I learned about the importance of including a diverse and flexible exercise routine into my daily life. The key was to remain open, considering my mood, seasons, weather conditions, and the opportunities available. Here is a glimpse into the variety of workouts that became an important part of my fitness journey:

1. Walking - Seizing Everyday Opportunities:

I maximized the benefits of walking by incorporating it into my daily routine. Whether it was parking a few blocks away from work or choosing to stroll through the neighborhood to only buy three tomatoes from the supermarket, every step contributed to my overall activity levels. I even used to go to the toilet downstairs instead of the one on the same level as my work office in order to maximize the number of steps I was taking daily.

2. Stair Climbing - Elevating My Routine:

Opting for stairs over elevators whenever possible became a simple yet effective way to integrate cardio into my day. This choice not only burned calories but also enhanced my cardiovascular fitness. Do this a few times and you will notice it becomes easier and you are faster every time.

3. Zumba - A Joyful Fitness Experience:

Attending local Zumba classes during the week and enjoying free classes by the beach on Sundays during summer brought a sense of joy to my fitness routine. The lively music and dynamic movements made the exercise feel like a celebration. It's so nice and motivating to see people of all ages, women and men, joining in for an hour of fun, music and dance.

4. **Running - Family Bonding in the Park:**
Running in the local park with my husband or children became a cherished family activity. It not only promoted cardiovascular health but also fostered a sense of unity and shared accomplishment. Recently we joined the parkrun movement which is a 5km run happening probably even in your local park, a free event, every Saturday at 8 am. Give it a go, you can even walk the 5km… Check this out: www.parkrun.com

5. **Dancing - A Solo Celebration:**
Dancing at home to Latino music from YouTube created a lively and enjoyable workout environment. It allowed me to express myself freely and burn calories while having lots of fun. Great alternative for rainy or cold or too hot weather when you do not feel like going out.

6. **Biking - Exploring Local Routes:**
Taking advantage of local bike rides, I explored nearby areas on two wheels. Occasionally venturing to a mountain bike park added an adventurous element to my fitness routine and it was also a great opportunity to bond with my son since we are the only ones in our family enjoying mountain biking.

7. **Football and Basketball - Active Family Time:**
Engaging in activities like kicking a ball in the park with my children or shooting hoops with a basketball added an element of fun and family bonding to my exercise routine. I really needed something a bit different from time to time

and I was happy to play the games of my childhood with my children.

8. Hiking - Nature-Inspired Fitness:

Whenever I had the opportunity, I sought out hiking trails during holidays or long weekend getaways. Connecting with nature while staying active became a rejuvenating aspect of my fitness journey. And there are so many in New Zealand, for any fitness level!

9. Gym - Utilizing Opportunities During Travel:

While I didn't have a gym membership at home, I made use of hotel gyms during holidays or city breaks. It allowed me to maintain my fitness routine even when away from home and again, it was something different from my normal routine. I now have a gym membership and I joined it to complete my strength training or cross-training during the days when I don't do my running.

10. Gardening and House Chores - Everyday Calorie Burn:

Recognizing that every movement counts, I embraced the calories burned through activities like gardening and house chores. Turning daily tasks into opportunities for physical activity became a holistic approach to staying active. Anything that helped me burn calories was great, so funnily enough, out of a sudden, I wasn't so upset anymore to clean up my home as it made me lose weight. What a new perspective! Even getting off the couch to bring someone in my family a glass of water was an opportunity to add more steps to the daily count. I know, it might sound like an exaggeration, but this change of perspective helped me immensely.

Staying Motivated and Consistent Is Key

To maintain motivation and consistency, I reminded myself that every form of movement contributed to my overall wellbeing. I celebrated the diversity of my workouts, allowing myself the freedom to choose activities based on my mood and circumstances. Additionally, involving my family and friends in some activities made exercise a shared experience, fostering a supportive and encouraging environment.

In the journey to a healthier lifestyle, the key was not just to exercise for weight loss but to find joy and fulfillment in the diverse range of physical activities. This approach helped me shed pounds and also transformed exercise into a sustainable and enjoyable part of my daily life.

Chapter Eight

Stick with these three daily practices for short and long-term weight loss success

In my experience, there are just three things that you have to religiously stick with day by day while trying to lose weight. So if you're looking to streamline your daily routine for effective weight loss, consider focusing on these three essential practices:

1. **Morning Weigh-In Ritual:** Begin your day by stepping onto the scale before consuming food or liquids. To ensure accuracy, it's beneficial to visit the toilet first, to eliminate any extra weight. This consistent morning weigh-in provides valuable data for tracking your progress and adjusting your approach as needed. Record your weight every day on your phone or in a journal.

2. **Record Your Meals:** Log every meal and snack meticulously, keeping a close eye on calorie intake. By maintaining a food diary, on your phone, in a Notepad App or in a notebook or journal, you gain a valuable awareness of your dietary choices, enabling better-informed decisions and accountability. This practice empowers you to align your eating habits with your weight loss goals, make adjustments, and improve your knowledge and experience.

3. **Exercise:** Incorporate daily exercise into your routine and measure the calories burned during each session. Whether it's a brisk walk, a workout at the gym, or a home-based exercise routine,

regular physical activity is integral to weight loss. Monitoring calories burned helps you understand the impact of your efforts and ensures a balanced approach to achieving a calorie deficit.

While sticking to these three practices can significantly contribute to your weight loss journey, it's important to acknowledge that perfection isn't the goal. There will be days when you forget to use the scale in the morning, exceed your planned calorie intake, or find it challenging to fit in a workout. Instead of dwelling on these occasional lapses, view them as normal fluctuations in your journey. The key is to avoid repetitive negative patterns and learn from each experience. Don't let minor setbacks derail your progress; instead, focus on consistency and commitment. By adopting this mindset, you empower yourself to navigate challenges with resilience and continue moving toward your weight loss goals.

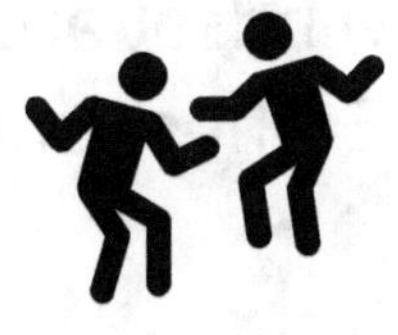

Chapter Nine

About My Mindset and Contagious Enthusiasm

My weight loss journey went beyond physical transformations for me; it went deeper into the complex realm of mental strength. Understanding the mental aspects of weight loss is crucial for setting realistic expectations, staying motivated, and overcoming the inevitable challenges that may arise along the way.

Setting Realistic Expectations

One of the cornerstones of a successful weight loss journey is establishing realistic expectations. Acknowledge that progress may not always follow a linear path – I learned this the hard way, and quick fixes are rarely sustainable. Consider setting achievable short-term goals (a SMART goal could be 5kgs in 3 months, remember?), celebrating small victories, and recognizing that true and lasting transformation takes time. This mindset shift not only requires patience, but also ensures that you appreciate the incremental changes that contribute to long-term success.

Staying Motivated

Maintaining motivation throughout your weight loss journey can be challenging, but it's an important factor in sustaining progress. Cultivate a positive mindset by focusing on the reasons behind your desire to lose weight – your WHY. One of my secret dreams was to replace all my clothes in my wardrobe. Cheeky. What other better reason one could have for losing weight than changing the whole wardrobe because there are no more clothes that would fit? Whether it's improved health, increased energy, or enhanced self-confidence, connecting with your deeper motivations can serve as a powerful anchor during moments of doubt. Find your WHY and always get back to it and re-connect. Additionally, vary your routines, try new exercises, and involve friends or family to make the process enjoyable and dynamic and get permanent support.

Strategies for Dealing with Challenges

Challenges are an inevitable part of any weight loss journey. When faced with obstacles, consider them as opportunities for growth rather than insurmountable roadblocks. If you encounter a setback, analyze its root cause without self-judgment, and use it as a learning experience. Be kind to yourself. Incorporate flexibility into your plan, recognizing that life's unpredictability may require adjustments. Seek support from friends, family, or a professional, as sharing your challenges can provide valuable perspectives and encouragement.

Overcoming Plateaus

Weight loss plateaus are very common and can be discouraging. Instead of letting them derail your progress, view plateaus as a natural phase in your journey. Reevaluate your habits, reassess your goals, and consider introducing new elements to your routine, such as varying your workouts or adjusting your calorie intake. Funnily, it's recommended that you increase your daily calories which may seem counterintuitive. Celebrate non-scale victories, like improved energy levels or clothing fitting better, or your skin looking brighter and healthier, to reinforce positive changes beyond the numbers on the scale. One of my bonus benefits during my weight loss journey was my improved skin appearance. I had no more pimples and my face looked so much cleaner and younger. I supposed this amazing and unexpected change was possible mainly because of the increased intake of fruits and vegetables and also reduced sugar and alcohol.

Mindful Self-Compassion

Throughout your weight loss journey, practice mindful self-compassion. Be kind to yourself, especially in moments of perceived failure like plateaus or lack of motivation. Understand that setbacks are temporary, and your worth is not defined by the number on the scale at that very moment. Cultivate a positive internal dialogue, focusing on self-love and appreciation for the efforts you invest in your wellbeing and for all the progress you've made.

I believe that a successful weight loss journey requires a robust mental framework. By setting realistic expectations, staying motivated, and developing strategies for overcoming challenges and plateaus, you enhance the likelihood of achieving your goals and also cultivate a resilient and positive mindset that extends beyond the scale. Remember, your journey is unique, and each step forward, no matter how small, is a triumph worth celebrating.

Cultivating Personal Appreciation and Embracing Your Unique Journey

In the realm of weight loss, it is vital to resist the temptation of comparing oneself to others. Each individual's journey is unique and influenced by a myriad of factors such as metabolism, genetics, and lifestyle. Constantly measuring one's progress against the achievements of others can lead to frustration and undermine the significance of personal accomplishments. Instead, I learned to appreciate my own journey by looking back at the progress I've made thus far. Reflecting on the effort invested and the positive changes achieved provided a more meaningful perspective. Acknowledging my achievements and focusing on my personal growth allowed me to cultivate a sense of self-appreciation, reinforcing the understanding that the journey towards a healthier lifestyle is deeply personal and unfolds at its own pace.

Inspiring Others: A Contagious Enthusiasm for Change

During my weight loss journey, I discovered that the enthusiasm for positive change is contagious. I wasn't only navigating the path to better health for myself, I actually became an example and an inspiration for my friends, my co-workers, and even my husband. The catalyst for this life-changing period was my total, 100% involvement in my weight loss project, a journey that not only reshaped my relationship with food, but also ignited a shared passion for wellness within my social circles.

Spreading the Noom Momentum

As I delved into the Noom program and witnessed its effectiveness in reshaping my habits, I couldn't help but share my newfound enthusiasm with those around me and even thousands of miles away. Friends and co-workers, inspired by my visible results and energized commitment, joined me on this health adventure. The new health approach, blending psychology with nutrition education and physical activity, resonated with many people, offering a sustainable way to lose weight that went beyond only calorie counting.

Leading by Example

Inevitably, my husband, initially skeptical but observant of my consistent progress, eventually became intrigued. Witnessing the positive changes in my life and acknowledging that I maintained my success over many months, he decided to try the program himself. My enthusiasm for healthier choices, coupled with this sustainable and holistic approach, was a testament to how effective the method was.

The beauty of this journey we went on together was not just in individual accomplishments but in shared triumphs and mutual encouragement. We exchanged tips, celebrated victories, and navigated challenges as a united front. The contagious enthusiasm reverberated through our support network, creating a positive and empowering environment that fuelled our collective commitment to lasting change.

Maintaining the Momentum

Months after achieving our initial goals, this new approach continued to be an integral part of our lives. The shared experiences and results reinforced the sustainability of this new weight loss method, turning healthy habits into a lifestyle. Our contagious enthusiasm evolved into a persistent commitment to long-term wellbeing, and the positive ripple effect extended far beyond the confines of a weight loss journey.

In the end, the contagious enthusiasm that started with my personal transformation became a catalyst for a broader movement toward health and wellness. It wasn't just about losing weight; it was about embracing a holistic lifestyle that inspired others to embark on their own life-changing journeys. The ripple effect of positivity and shared commitment showed how our commitment can really make a big difference in the overall journey towards wellbeing.

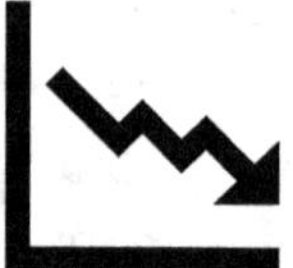

Chapter Ten

Tracking Progress

I monitor my progress by daily hopping on the scale and recording my weight. Logging my food in the app helped me monitor my calorie intake but also the quality of my meals. Noom has a special system that encourages the consumption of fruit and vegetables and moderate consumption of the other food categories. This is when I realised that even though I was eating a good variety of foods, there was a bit too much full-fat dairy or red meat or even nuts, olive oil or avocados in my daily meals. The sweet stuff also represented a relatively large proportion of my meals, especially in the form of snacks. So I figured out I could prioritize eating fruit and only if I was still craving some dessert, I could have it. To cut down on calories but keep the same delicious foods in my diet. For instance I started eating less cheese and experimenting with drinking low-fat milk. Soon I had the big surprise that this move or the slight change of diet made me get bloated less often and my skin, especially my face, looked spotless. No more the odd pimple! No more bloating every day!

During this amazing journey, I discovered new recipes, I re-discovered the beauty and the simplicity of basic, nutritious food like raw fruits and vegetables, salads with simple dressings, lean meats without too complicated sauces, the roughness and the rich taste of wholemeal and wholegrain pasta, rice or bread and so on.

So both the daily weigh-in and the food logging helped me not only keep track of my progress and adjust my strategy and diet according to my findings but also re-invent the way I ate and what I ate.

Consequently, I felt better physically relatively shortly after I started my weight loss journey and I found myself captivated by the thrilling appeal of rediscovery and an unknown future, filled with pleasant surprises.

Planning and preparing your meals in advance is key

Having said that, a valuable lesson I learned was that planning my meals was key to staying on track. I almost always had a plan around my breakfast and my lunch and not only that but I prepared them a day in advance or had all the ingredients ready for the next day. These were the times when I was the busiest and there was a high risk of eating more or inappropriate food or going starving because of lack of choices which would later lead to food binging.

I had a mission, I had a goal, I had a strategy and successful tactics and I was determined to apply all of them to get to the finish line. Sharing every step of my journey with my family and friends also helped a lot because that kept me accountable and motivated.

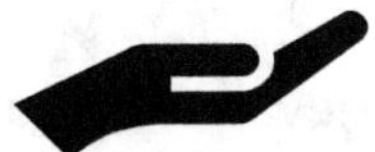

Chapter Eleven

Embracing Support and Accountability

My weight loss journey was a wonderful experience for me that often required more than just my personal determination. One of the essential factors contributing to a successful and sustainable weight loss project is the support and accountability provided by friends, family, and even work colleagues or dedicated support groups. The Noom app has a forum that connects you with similar weight loss champions across the world. There you can share your experience and ask questions. The main gain from this is that you see that you are not alone, many others like you have success, have difficulties, and have good and bad days. There are celebrations and encouragements and this support means the world in these moments. In this chapter, I'll tell you how my different support groups worked and we'll explore the significant role these connections play in your journey and create strategies for finding the right partners to accompany you on this transformative path.

The Power of Support Systems

1. Family Dynamics:

Your family can serve as a crucial pillar of support in your weight loss journey. When you're lucky enough to have family members like me who are not only supportive but also actively interested in your progress, it can significantly enhance your motivation. Share your daily lessons, tips, tricks, and challenges with them. Find foods that you can eat and share with them. Alter the food you are already eating so it can work for you, but also make everyone's meals healthier. Join them for walks or the sports they do or challenge them to follow you and move more during the day and the weekends. Their understanding and encouragement can be instrumental in keeping you on track.

2. Friendship Across Distances:

Friends, whether near or far, can play an integral role in your weight loss journey. Technology has made it easier than ever to stay connected, enabling friends from different locations to share in your experience. I set up a WhatsApp group with my best friends and we shared recipes, pictures, progress and also my difficult days. We had also a weekly call where we caught up about what happened in the last week and shared all the latest learnings. Your friends' curiosity and willingness to stay updated on your progress can create a sense of accountability and camaraderie that fosters motivation. This was definitely what helped me immensely. One of my friends from overseas also started the program at some point during my journey. Her progress made me so happy and determined to achieve my goals and also help other people. Something was working and I was eager to share my experience and show my friends that there is hope and I have discovered something sustainable, long term and practically a new, healthy lifestyle.

3. Joining the Journey:

The impact of having my friends join me on my weight loss journey cannot be overstated. The shared experience not only strengthened my support system but also provided a platform for mutual encouragement and celebration of victories, no matter how small. My little WhatsApp group of BFFs transformed my weight loss journey from a solo effort into a collective pursuit of finding and living a healthy lifestyle.

How to Find Accountability Partners

1. Transparent Communication:
Seek individuals who are willing to engage in open and honest communication about your goals. Share your expectations, struggles, and achievements, creating an environment where accountability is fostered through understanding.

2. Similar Goals and Values:
Look for partners who share similar weight loss goals or values related to health and wellness. Shared objectives create a common ground that strengthens the commitment to supporting one another.

3. Professional Guidance:
In some cases, professional guidance may be necessary. Consider consulting with a nutritionist, fitness trainer, or weight loss coach. These experts can provide personalized advice and structured plans, adding a layer of accountability through regular check-ins and assessments.

Cultivating Motivation through Sharing

1. Blogging or Journaling:
Consider documenting your journey through a blog or journal. Sharing your experiences publicly not only holds you accountable but also inspires others who may be on a similar path. The feedback and support you receive can be a powerful motivator. I didn't do this to document my weight loss journey, but more recently when I started another chapter of my life which was running in competitions and training for them, I discovered the power of logging my progress and sharing my daily feelings and thoughts about how my runs and workouts went. I felt like at the end of the day those moments of journaling helped me solidify my progress, and my determination and

re-fuel my motivation to continue. Those were also the moments when I could express my gratitude for my mind that guided me along this adventure and for my body that listened to my mind, carried me, and propelled me through these amazingly challenging but rewarding days.

2. Social Media Engagement:

Leverage the power of social media to connect with a larger community. Join weight loss groups, share your progress, and engage with others who are on similar journeys. The virtual support network can provide encouragement and valuable insights. Again I did not use social media that extensively during my weight loss journey apart from sharing my biggest milestones with my close friends. I guess my support system formed by my family, close friends, and work colleagues plus the forum on the Noom app was enough to offer me a great platform to grow and lean on. However, more recently, when my running adventure took off, I discovered the many Facebook groups that shared the same goals and went through the same challenges as me - related to running and, in particular, half marathons. There was a wealth of information shared, a lot of celebrations and victories made public, and many questions asked which answers I was interested in or maybe even able to answer from my own experience. Of course, take everything with a grain of salt and try filtering with what is an opinion, a personal experience or a piece of more professional advice. However the vibes and the support I found in those groups are exceptional and those groups are definitely worth exploring.

In conclusion, the support and accountability you cultivate on your weight loss journey can make all the difference in your success. Whether it's the fantastic encouragement of family, the virtual camaraderie of friends, or the expertise of professionals, these connections provide the foundation upon which your transformation rests. Embrace these relationships, share your story, and let the collective strength of your support system propel you toward your health and wellness goals.

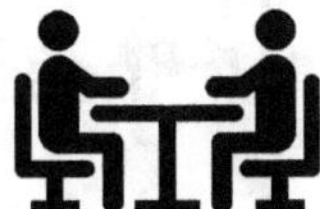

Chapter Twelve

Harnessing Workplace Support for Holistic Wellness

In the complex world of weight loss, where determination generates transformation, the workplace can become a surprising yet potent ally. I am again lucky enough to work for a small company where my colleagues are like a big family to me. So I shared my weight loss journey from the first day and they embraced it as I did. My work colleagues, with their shared routines and mutual understanding, not only provided an additional layer of support, apart from family and friends but also became active participants in the narrative of my personal journey. My new healthier lifestyle and my great connection to my work colleagues led to an important event in my work life too. This was the culmination of the wellness journey I am currently on. It started with my idea that my workplace needed more concrete and moral support to thrive, to grow and to become even more connected with each other. The main goal was to come to work with pleasure, do a great job, feel good about building a good life for yourself and contributing to the business, and leave work at the end of the day with a smile on your face and happy to come back the next day. In more corporate words my Happiness Program objectives were: employee engagement, stress reduction, enhanced productivity, positive work culture, rewards and recognition, health and wellness, purpose and meaning, retention and recruitment. A couple of years ago I became the Chief Happiness Officer, one of the best moments in my career!

Let's explore the unique role my workplace played in my holistic approach to weight loss. You might find something useful that you can apply to your own work environment.

1. Workplace Camaraderie:
My colleagues, like an extended family, played a pivotal role in my journey. Their genuine interest, support, and enthusiasm added a layer of friendship that transcended professional boundaries. Sharing my daily experiences with them created a positive, inspirational and motivating atmosphere within the workplace.

2. Collective Empowerment:
The decision of two other colleagues to join the weight loss program speaks volumes about the contagious nature of my enthusiasm. The amazing empowerment that came out of this shared commitment not only strengthened my determination but also fostered a sense of unity and positive support among us as coworkers.

3. Mutual Learning and Celebrations:
The beauty of having colleagues on a similar journey lies in the exchange of insights and unique experiences almost every day. Each person's approach and discoveries added a valuable layer of learning, making the weight loss process richer and more dynamic. I felt I was losing weight and winning friends. We were also sharing an amazing present and winning a healthier future. Celebrating successes together created a culture of continuous encouragement. I don't even know if we realized all this then. I'm so grateful for my colleagues and their support!

4. Integrating Physical Activity:

The holistic nature of my weight loss method, incorporating not only dietary changes but also a focus on gym, sports, or other physical activities, underscores a comprehensive approach to wellbeing. The workplace became a hub for promoting an active and healthy lifestyle. We went to Zumba classes, took longer walks, and engaged our families in more active weekends.

5. Encouraging a Holistic Lifestyle:
The combination of healthy eating and physical activity within the workplace showcased a commitment to holistic wellness. My colleagues went to cooking classes, went to chiropractors to fix their ailments, and visited nutritionists to help themselves and their family members. This approach, beyond mere weight loss, fosters overall health, resilience, and a positive work environment.

6. Group Motivation:
The shared commitment of colleagues amplifies motivation. Knowing that you are not alone in your journey and having a group of like-minded individuals rooting for each other creates a powerful motivational force. That was 100% my case. The workplace became a hub for mutual encouragement, transforming it into a supportive community which I am very grateful for.

7. Translating Success Beyond the Scale:
The holistic approach to weight loss, extending beyond the scale to encompass broader lifestyle changes, mirrors a sustainable and balanced philosophy. This mindset, cultivated within my workplace, had the potential to influence not only individual wellbeing but also the overall culture of the organization.

How to Foster a Supportive Workplace Culture

1. Wellness Programs:
Encourage workplace wellness programs that promote both physical and mental health. These initiatives can include fitness challenges, nutritional workshops, or even mindfulness sessions.

2. Open Dialogue:
Foster open dialogue about health and wellness within the workplace. Creating a culture where colleagues feel comfortable sharing their journeys and goals contributes to a supportive environment.

3. Team-building Activities:
Organize team-building activities that incorporate physical fitness. This not only promotes a healthy lifestyle but also strengthens bonds among colleagues.

4. Recognizing Achievements:
Acknowledge and celebrate achievements related to health and wellness. This recognition reinforces the importance of wellbeing and encourages others to embark on their journeys.

In summary, the workplace formed a dynamic and supportive backdrop for my weight loss journey. It could do that for you too. Be the change in your workplace! The shared commitment, mutual encouragement, and integration of holistic wellness practices transformed my workplace into a hub of positivity and wellbeing. Embrace this supportive culture, share your journey, and inspire others to jump on their opportunities toward a healthier

and more balanced life. You will be amazed by the change
you will see in others.

Chapter Thirteen

Navigating Challenges on the Weight Loss Journey

The path to weight loss is often peppered with challenges that test our willpower and determination. In this chapter, we'll explore common obstacles I faced during my fantastic journey and share practical strategies to overcome them. By understanding and addressing these hurdles, you can strengthen your commitment to a healthier lifestyle.

Cravings and How to Conquer the Food Temptations

<u>Challenge:</u>
Cravings can be relentless, threatening to derail even the most disciplined eater like me. I am very disciplined, but when it comes to certain desserts I can be defeated. So whether it's the allure of sweets, the comfort of savoury snacks, or the siren call of indulgent treats, cravings can be a formidable foe.

<u>Solution:</u>
- **Mindful Eating:** Pause and reflect on your cravings. Are they triggered by hunger, emotions, or habits? Understanding the root cause helps in making healthier choices.

- **Healthy Alternatives:** Identify satisfying alternatives to curb cravings. Opt for a piece of dark chocolate (over 70%, the darker the better), a handful of nuts (not too many though and not covered in chocolate or yogurt coating), or fresh fruit to satiate your sweet tooth in a more wholesome way.

- **Hydration:** Sometimes, cravings are a signal of dehydration. Drink a glass of water before reaching for a snack to ensure your body isn't misinterpreting thirst as hunger. This worked for me 80% of the time!

Social Situations and How to Navigate the Feast and Festivities

<u>Challenge:</u>
Social gatherings and celebrations often revolve around food (fortunately or not), making it challenging to stick to a weight loss plan. But there are plenty of ways around this.

<u>Solution:</u>
- **Plan Ahead:** If possible, review the menu before going to a restaurant or attending an event. Choose healthier options and plan your portions to avoid impulsive decisions.

- **Mindful Indulgence:** Allow yourself to enjoy special treats in moderation. It's not worth refraining from something that you really like. But do not eat anything if you don't want to. You can say no to your hosts and don't feel bad about doing that. Actually you should feel good about your determination. Acknowledge that most of the time at parties or gatherings we eat just because everyone else does. We are not hungry. So instead, make sure you savour each bite, and be conscious of your choices without feeling deprived.

- **Communication:** Inform friends and family about your weight loss journey. Their support and understanding can help create an environment that aligns with your goals.

Time Constraints: Balancing Work, Life, and Wellness

<u>Challenge:</u>
Busy schedules and time constraints can make it challenging to prioritize healthy eating and regular exercise.

<u>Solution:</u>
- **Meal Prep:** Dedicate time to plan and prepare meals in advance. This is rule number 1 and it was life-saving for me! Having healthy, portioned options readily available reduces reliance on convenient, but often less nutritious, alternatives. Prepare breakfast and work lunch the night before.

- **Short, Intense Workouts:** Opt for shorter, high-intensity workouts. They can be just as effective as longer sessions and are easier to fit into a busy schedule. At the beginning of my weight loss program, I went to the gym three times a week for an hour each time. I did it for a while but it felt very time-consuming and at some point, I was not looking forward to it. So I reduced the gym visits to 30 min each. Surprisingly they were as effective as the 1-hour ones.

- **Schedule Prioritization:** Recognize the importance of self-care. Schedule workouts, meal times, meditation, and even massages as non-negotiable appointments, treating them with the same importance as work meetings.

Plateaus and How to Overcome Stagnation in Progress

<u>Challenge</u>:
Experiencing plateaus in weight loss can be disheartening, leaving one feeling stuck and demotivated. However, they do happen and even quite a few times during a three-month journey like mine. Don't despair, just treat them as normal. They will pass. They're part of the process.

<u>Solution</u>:
- **Ride the Waves:** When the scale seems resistant to change for a few weeks, take a moment to inhale deeply. Stay resilient, and resist the urge to make impulsive changes. Simply remain patient and ride the waves. Just because the scale hits a pause doesn't mean there are errors in your approach. Throughout your weight loss journey, you are consistently cultivating habits that will last a lifetime, progressing steadily towards your goals. A lack of weight loss doesn't equate to a lack of progress. You are still adhering to your healthy habits; it's just that the scale might not reflect it at this precise moment. And it's quite frustrating, I know. Trust the process.

- **Diversify Workouts:** Introduce variety into your exercise routine. This can shock your body into responding positively and break through the plateau.

- **Reevaluate Diet:** Periodically reassess your dietary habits. Are you inadvertently consuming more calories than you think? Adjust portion sizes and reassess nutritional choices if this is the case.

- **Increase your calorie intake:** What? You will be surprised to hear that sometimes you will need to increase your daily calorie amount to rev up your metabolism. I was puzzled to realize that I was doing everything by the book, watching and tracking my meals and calorie intake, doing at least 10000 steps every day, doing other physical activities as well, having a good sleep, and keeping my stress under control and still my weight loss stopped. For days, the program told me that that was normal and that increasing the calories I eat would solve the problem in the short term. Research findings documented in the International Journal of Obesity and Related Metabolic Disorders, the American Journal of Clinical Nutrition, and other publications indicate that engaging in "overfeeding" – wherein one increases their calorie intake after a period of calorie deficit – can lead to heightened feelings of satisfaction and an immediate boost in calorie expenditure. Wow! Try it, it's so rewarding! I love science and I love experiments so if you are like me, you will be so excited to try this.

- **Eat more protein:** For instance, increasing protein intake can help reverse a weight loss stall by boosting metabolism, reducing hunger and preventing muscle mass loss.

- **Eat more fiber:** Fiber promotes weight loss by slowing the movement of food through your digestive tract, decreasing appetite and reducing the number of calories your body absorbs from food.

- **Celebrate Non-Scale Victories:** This is very important. Plateaus aren't solely measured on the scale. Celebrate other victories, such as improved stamina, better-looking skin, increased energy levels, or clothing fitting better.

By addressing these common obstacles with practical solutions, you'll be better equipped to overcome challenges on your weight loss journey. Remember, the path to a healthier you is not linear and always smooth, but with resilience and strategic planning, you can navigate any hurdle that comes your way.

Chapter Fourteen

My Remarkable Lifestyle Changes and How They Have Helped Me

Going on this weight loss journey was not just about shedding kilograms; it's been a profound transformation of my whole lifestyle. In this chapter, I'll talk about the most important lifestyle changes that contributed to my successful weight loss journey.

1. Quality Sleep and Power of Rest

<u>What I changed:</u>
Improved sleep was a cornerstone of my weight loss journey. Recognizing the impact of quality rest on overall health, I prioritized a consistent sleep schedule. Creating a tranquil bedtime routine and optimizing my sleep environment became very important in fostering both physical and mental wellbeing.

<u>Concrete Tips:</u>
1. I stick to a regular 8-9 hour sleep every day and go to sleep at the same time every day even during weekends. I also try to wake up at the same time every day even during weekends.
2. I read a few pages almost every night before sleep and this makes the transition from the living room to my bedroom and from a full, energetic day to a quiet night.
3. I practice meditation and I make a small prayer. I use the Balance app for my guided meditations which is a fantastic tool, very useful and diversified. I usually fall asleep during my sleep meditation. I'm so relaxed...

4. Take naps, they are unbelievable energy boosters. I feel so much more energized after an afternoon nap and I usually go for a run or a long walk afterwards.

<u>Why It Matters:</u>
Adequate sleep regulates hunger hormones, supports metabolism, and enhances energy levels. By optimizing my sleep patterns, I harnessed a rejuvenated body and mind for the challenges and successes of each day.

2. Stress Management and Why It Is a Balancing Act

<u>What I changed:</u>
Stress, once a terrible enemy, transformed into a manageable aspect of my life. Incorporating stress management techniques such as mindfulness, deep breathing, self-care and periodic breaks allowed me to navigate challenges with resilience.

<u>Concrete Tips:</u>
1. Stop using your phone or watching TV when you eat. If you are alone, focus on your meal, the texture, the colors, the taste of different ingredients and how amazingly they blend on the plate and then in your mouth. If you have company, enjoy a pleasant conversation and a shared meal. Food is better when shared.
2. Practice deep breathing and meditation even during the day when you feel your stress level is rising.
3. A self-massage, a face mask or a short walk outdoors can quickly restore your calm.

4. Use the Pomodoro technique if you want to be more productive at work or at home and let your colleagues or family know you cannot be interrupted. The Pomodoro Technique is a time management method developed by Francesco Cirillo. It involves breaking your work into intervals, traditionally 25 minutes in length, separated by short, 5 minute breaks. These intervals are known as "pomodoros". After completing four pomodoros, you take a longer break. This technique is designed to enhance focus, productivity, and efficiency by leveraging the benefits of focused work sessions and regular breaks.

<u>Why It Matters:</u>
Chronic stress can hinder weight loss progress. By embracing effective stress management, I not only gained a calmer mindset but also created an environment encouraging healthier choices and consistent personal growth.

3. Breaking Unhealthy Habits and How I Felt Liberated

<u>What I Changed:</u>
Identifying and breaking free from unhealthy habits was a great ride in itself. Whether it was mindless snacking, emotional eating, or sedentary behaviors, I adopted conscious choices that aligned with my wellness goals.

<u>Concrete Tips:</u>
1. I started counting the almonds I ate. I snacked on 10 almonds not half of a little container at my desk

during my work. Count 10 and put the rest away. Apparently an almond amounts to 7 calories, so I guess 70 calories as a snack was fine. I was eating them mindlessly anyway.

2. I now recognize when I eat because I am bored or I do routine, repetitive work. Like checking emails. Instead of reaching into my drawer where I keep healthy snacks, I get up and I go for a cup of tea or to fill my water bottle. I make sure I say hi and exchange a few words with the colleagues I meet on my way.

3. There is no way I do not do something physical every day. 10000 steps is my general goal. Try and include a walk, a run, work in the garden, or anything that gets you moving. My day is not complete if I don't tick the workout box every day. A small thing is better than nothing.

<u>Why It Matters:</u>
Unhealthy habits are stumbling blocks on the path to weight loss. By replacing them with mindful choices, I created a sustainable and positive relationship with food, exercise, and overall wellbeing. I put myself first.

4. Physical Activity Integration in My Life and How It Redefined Me

<u>What I Changed:</u>
Exercise ceased to be a chore; it became an integral part of my lifestyle. I embraced activities that brought joy, whether it was walking, running, dancing, hiking, going to the gym, or engaging in Zumba classes. Making movement enjoyable and diverse was key to consistency.

<u>Concrete Tips:</u>
1. Join a local Zumba or any fitness class or a running club. It makes a big difference to meet people like you regularly and have fun together. My Zumba classes kept me committed and even if one day I was not in the mood to go, I didn't want to let my friends and instructor down. I never regretted going to a class, it was so much fun every time.
2. I often call a friend when I walk and even when I run slow. I feel so accomplished doing two great things at the same time, connecting with a friend and catching up and staying fit.
3. When I come home from work, I get changed in my workout clothes. It's easier and straightforward to get out the door and I also don't feel like sitting on the couch wearing my active outfit.

<u>Why It Matters:</u>
Regular physical activity is not just about burning calories; it's a celebration of what our bodies can achieve. I started loving my body even more, and not only because it looked better but also because it did so much for me. By finding activities I loved, I fostered a long-lasting commitment to a more active lifestyle.

5. Nutrient-Rich Eating and How I Discovered Food Was a Joy

<u>What I Changed:</u>
Dietary changes were not about deprivation – wow, I love Noom for making me realize that - but about nourishing my body. I shifted towards a diet rich in whole foods, incorporating a colorful array of fruits, vegetables, lean proteins, and whole grains.

<u>Concrete Tips:</u>

1. I knew about how nutrient-dense wholemeal pasta and bread could be compared to white pasta and white bread but I started being more consistent in stocking my pantry with them and eating them. I also added way more brown rice to my diet and ditched the white one.
2. I started eating more fruit and more salads. I found new salad recipes that combined vegetables and fruits and protein and that was my lunch most of the time.
3. By preparing my own food and choosing basic ingredients to make my meals, I realized I ate less sugar and less processed food. I re-discovered the pleasure of eating raw food, simple and homemade meals. I also started gardening which provided my family with organic vegetables and fruit. And to be honest, there was not much room left for other types of food.

<u>Why It Matters:</u>

Nourishing my body with nutrient-dense foods fuelled my energy, supported my workouts, and contributed to sustainable weight loss. It was a culinary revolution that made me embrace the joy of wholesome, delicious, homemade, shared meals.

In essence, these lifestyle changes were not only adjustments; they were profound shifts that solidified my commitment to a healthier and more fulfilling life. Through prioritizing quality sleep, managing stress effectively, breaking free from unhealthy habits, embracing enjoyable physical activities, and savouring nutrient-rich foods, I created a lifestyle that supported my weight loss journey and also became the foundation of my holistic and sustainable wellbeing.

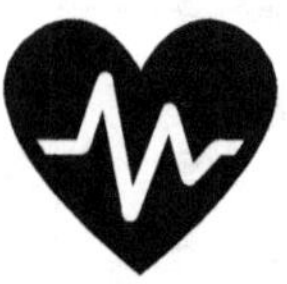

Chapter Fifteen

Prioritizing Health and Safety on Your Weight Loss Journey

When you depart on a weight loss journey you make a great decision but this requires careful consideration and a commitment to your wellbeing. In this chapter, I will talk about the crucial aspects of health and safety during the weight loss process. It is imperative to prioritize sustainable and healthy methods while keeping a vigilant eye on your mental health and overall wellbeing.

The Importance of Healthy and Sustainable Weight Loss

Before digging into the intricacies of weight loss, it is crucial to understand that the goal is not just shedding pounds rapidly but creating a new, sustainable, and healthier lifestyle. Rapid weight loss methods may yield short-term results, but they often come at the expense of your health and they usually don't have lasting results. You need to embrace the idea that a gradual, steady approach is not only effective but also significantly safer for your body.

Consulting Healthcare Professionals

One of the foundational steps in any weight loss journey should be consulting with healthcare professionals, especially if you have a history of health issues. Prioritize scheduling a comprehensive medical check-up before embarking on any significant lifestyle changes. A thorough examination and comprehensive blood tests can help identify any underlying health conditions and deficiencies, ensuring that your weight loss plan aligns with your overall wellbeing.

Before my own weight loss journey, I visited with my family doctor and made sure my body was functioning properly and it was ready for a challenge. For some people, seeing even a registered dietitian might be a great idea. They can provide valuable insights into your unique health profile, helping tailor a weight loss plan that addresses your specific needs. Having a personalized approach could make you feel more confident in the changes you will be making, knowing they are aligned with your overall health goals.

Safety Precautions

Safety should be at the forefront of your weight loss efforts. Incorporate safety measures into your plan to minimize the risk of injury or adverse effects. If your weight loss plan includes physical activity, start with activities that match your fitness level and gradually increase intensity. This gradual progression reduces the risk of strain or injury.

For instance what I learned, in the hard way, from my running experience, is that I need to take extra care before and after the workout to make sure my body is warmed up and cools down properly to avoid long-term, annoying injuries.

Here are some tips:

To prevent injury before a run, initiate a thorough **pre-run routine**:

- Begin with dynamic stretching, focusing on leg swings and lunges to enhance flexibility.

- Perform joint mobilization exercises to increase joint flexibility.
- Use a foam roller to release muscle tension.
- Incorporate activation exercises targeting the core and stabilizing muscles.
- Warm up gradually with light cardio, ensuring proper hydration and nutrition for energy.

After your run:
- Transition into a cool-down phase by gradually slowing your pace and finishing with brisk walking.
- Engage in static stretching for major muscle groups, holding each stretch to improve flexibility.
- Rehydrate and refuel with a mix of carbohydrates and protein to support muscle recovery.
- Utilize foam rolling and self-massage to alleviate muscle tension, followed by light strengthening exercises targeting potential weak areas.
- Listen to your body, addressing any signs of fatigue or discomfort promptly, and seek professional advice if needed.

Consistency in these routines contributes to injury prevention, promoting a sustainable and healthy running practice.

Additionally, stay well-hydrated every day even if you don't exercise, and maintain a balanced diet based on your physical activity levels, ensuring you're meeting your nutritional needs. Rapid or extreme changes in diet can lead to nutrient deficiencies, affecting your energy levels and overall health, so stay alert for any signals your body gives you.

Monitoring Progress Safely

Tracking progress is an integral part of any weight loss journey, but it should be done in a way that promotes positive habits and doesn't compromise your mental or physical health. Avoid fixating solely on the number on the scale, as weight fluctuations are natural. Focus on other indicators of progress, such as improved energy levels, better sleep, and enhanced mood.

As you navigate your weight loss journey, remember that the destination is not just a number on the scale but a sustainable and healthier lifestyle. Prioritize your health and safety by consulting with healthcare professionals, incorporating safety precautions, and monitoring your progress in a balanced manner. A holistic approach ensures that your journey is not only successful but also one that contributes positively to your whole life.

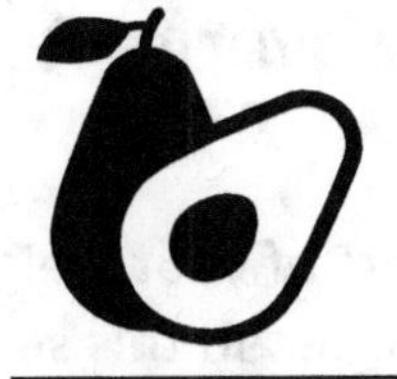

Chapter Sixteen

My Favorite Recipes

Welcome to the heart of your weight loss journey – "My Favorite Recipes" chapter. In this section, I will embark on a delightful exploration of my own nutritious and flavorful dishes meticulously crafted to support your health and fitness goals. These recipes are not just about counting calories; they're a celebration of the vibrant, delicious, and satisfying meals that can be an integral part of your sustainable weight loss journey. Whether you're a culinary enthusiast or a novice in the kitchen, these recipes are designed to make healthy eating an enjoyable and fulfilling experience. Get ready to savor every bite, as we will transform ordinary ingredients into extraordinary meals that nourish both body and soul, proving that weight loss can be a delicious and colorful, vibrant adventure, not a dull, boring one.

QUICK AND YUMMY BREAKFASTS

Eggs with Avocado and Tomato

Ingredients:
- 1 slice of wholemeal bread
- 1/2 ripe avocado, sliced
- 1 medium-sized tomato, sliced
- 1 large egg, scrambled or poached
- Salt and black pepper to taste
- Optional: Fresh herbs such as cilantro or chives for garnish

Instructions:
Prepare the Egg:

- Poach or scramble the egg using a non-stick cooking spray or a very small amount of olive oil. Season with salt and black pepper to taste.

Toast your bread slice.

Add the Egg:

- Spoon the scrambled or poached egg onto the bread slice.

Season and Garnish:

- Add your tomato and avocado
- Sprinkle a bit more salt and black pepper over everything.

Optionally, garnish with fresh herbs like cilantro or chives for added flavor.

Enjoy!

Your Egg, Avocado and Tomato Breakfast is ready to be enjoyed! It's a satisfying and low-calorie option rich in fiber, healthy fats, and protein. This breakfast is not only delicious but also provides a good balance of nutrients to keep you energized throughout the morning. The healthy fats from avocado, combined with the protein from the egg, make for a satisfying and nutritious start to your day. Feel free to customize this with additional veggies or herbs based on your preferences.

Chia Seed Pudding

Ingredients:

- 2 tablespoons chia seeds
- 1/2 cup unsweetened almond milk (or any milk of your choice)
- 1/4 teaspoon vanilla extract
- 1 teaspoon honey or maple syrup (optional, adjust to taste)

- Fresh berries for topping (strawberries, blueberries, raspberries)
- Mint leaves for garnish (optional)

<u>Instructions:</u>

Mix Chia Seeds and Liquid:

- In a bowl or a jar, combine chia seeds, almond milk, vanilla extract, and honey (if using). Stir well to ensure the chia seeds are evenly distributed.

Stir Again After 5 Minutes:

- After the initial mix, stir the chia seed mixture again after about 5 minutes. This prevents the chia seeds from clumping together.

Refrigerate Overnight:

- Cover the bowl or jar and refrigerate the mixture overnight or for at least 4-6 hours. The chia seeds will absorb the liquid and create a pudding-like consistency.

Check and Adjust Consistency:

- Before serving, check the consistency. If the pudding is too thick, you can add a little more almond milk and stir until you reach the desired thickness.

Top with Fresh Berries:

- Just before serving, top the chia seed pudding with fresh berries. Berries are low in calories and add a burst of flavor and nutrition.

Garnish (Optional):

- Garnish with mint leaves for a refreshing touch.

Enjoy Your Low-Calorie Breakfast:

- Dive into your delicious and low-calorie chia seed pudding! It's a nutrient-packed breakfast that provides a good source of fiber, omega-3 fatty acids, and antioxidants.

Feel free to customize this recipe by adding a sprinkle of cinnamon, a dollop of Greek yogurt, or a handful of sliced almonds for extra texture and flavor. This chia seed pudding is not only satisfying but also a great option for those looking to enjoy a tasty, low-calorie breakfast.

SALADS FOR LUNCH AS THE MAIN MEAL

Greek Salad Recipe

Ingredients:
- 1 cup cucumber, sliced or diced
- 1 cup tomatoes, diced
- 1 green/red/yellow bell pepper, chopped
- ¼ cup red onion, thinly sliced
- ¼ cup Kalamata olives, pitted
- 50g feta cheese, crumbled or diced
- 1 tablespoon extra-virgin olive oil
- 1 tablespoon apple cider vinegar
- 1 teaspoon dried oregano
- Salt and black pepper to taste

Instructions:
Prepare the Vegetables:
- Chop the cucumber, tomatoes, and bell pepper into bite-sized pieces.
- Thinly slice the red onion.
Assemble the Salad:

- In a large salad bowl, combine the diced cucumber, tomatoes, red onion, Kalamata olives, and chopped bell pepper.

Add Feta Cheese:

- Crumble or dice the feta cheese over the vegetables. The creamy texture of feta adds a rich and savory element to the salad.

Prepare the Dressing:

- In a small bowl, mix together the extra-virgin olive oil, vinegar, dried oregano, salt, and black pepper. Adjust the seasoning according to your taste preferences.

Dress the Salad:

- Drizzle the dressing over the salad ingredients. Gently toss the salad to ensure even coating.

Enjoy!

You could serve the Greek salad as a refreshing side dish or add grilled chicken or shrimp for a complete and satisfying dinner meal.

This Greek salad is a vibrant medley of colors and flavors, providing a healthy and delightful addition to your weight loss journey. Enjoy the freshness of crisp vegetables, the brininess of olives, and the creamy goodness of feta in every bite!

Roasted Vegetable Salad

<u>Ingredients:</u>

- 2 cups mixed vegetables, such as cherry tomatoes, bell peppers, zucchini, red onion, and carrots, potatoes, pumpkin, cut into bite-sized pieces

- 2 tablespoons olive oil
- 1 teaspoon dried thyme
- 1 teaspoon dried rosemary
- Salt and black pepper to taste
- 1 cup mixed salad greens (lettuce, spinach, arugula, etc.)
- 2 tablespoons balsamic vinaigrette dressing (olive oil, vinegar, salt)
- 50g crumbled feta cheese (optional)
- ¼ cup chopped fresh basil or parsley (optional, for garnish)

Instructions:

Preheat the Oven: Preheat your oven to 400°F (200°C).

Prepare Vegetables:

- In a large mixing bowl, toss the mixed vegetables with olive oil, dried thyme, dried rosemary, salt, and black pepper until well coated.

Roast Vegetables:

- Spread the seasoned vegetables in a single layer on a baking sheet lined with parchment paper.
- Roast in the preheated oven for about 20-25 minutes or until the vegetables are tender and slightly caramelized. Stir halfway through for even cooking.

Assemble the Salad:

- In a large salad bowl, combine the roasted vegetables with mixed salad greens.
- Add Feta Cheese: Sprinkle crumbled feta cheese over the roasted vegetables and salad greens.
- Drizzle with Dressing: Drizzle balsamic vinaigrette dressing over the salad. Adjust the amount according to your taste preference.

- Toss Gently: Toss the salad gently to combine all the ingredients, ensuring the dressing evenly coats the roasted vegetables and greens.

Garnish and Serve:

If desired, garnish the salad with chopped fresh basil or parsley for an extra burst of flavor and freshness.

You can serve warm or cold: Serve the roasted vegetable salad immediately for a warm dish, or refrigerate for a few hours to enjoy it cold.

This Roasted Vegetable Salad is not only delicious but also packed with nutrients and flavors. The combination of caramelized veggies, creamy feta, and a tangy balsamic dressing creates a satisfying and wholesome salad that can be enjoyed as a side dish or a light main course.

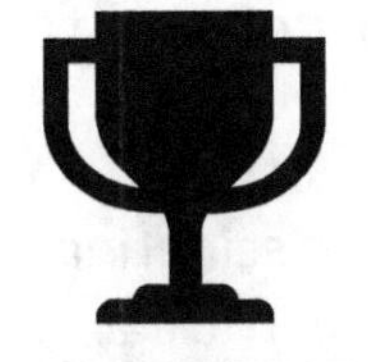

Chapter Seventeen

Success Stories

Probably my story is fascinating, but wait until you hear Megan's or Bogdan's or Tricia's.

Viewing Food as Fuel

Meet Megan – not just my colleague but a cherished friend, with our desks located a mere two meters apart. There's a saying that happiness is contagious, and indeed, the infectious quality of joy can set off a positive feedback loop. In our close proximity, the ripple effect of positivity is undeniable.

As I explored the workings of a new weight loss concept, my daily little stories, learnings, revelations, victories, and even the occasional setbacks became as contagious as germs, and Megan couldn't help but catch the enthusiasm that I shared.

Megan stood out as the most enthusiastic weight loss companion I've ever had. Her discipline and curiosity were unparalleled, and she wholeheartedly embraced the entire experience, a commitment that undoubtedly played a great role in her success. What set her apart even more was her active contribution to our journey – she shared her own insights, and interpretations, and recommended books that enriched our collective knowledge and made our shared experience exceptionally rich and special.

Here is what she has to say about her own experience:

"I've always struggled with my weight. The problem of finding a sustainable way to maintain a healthy weight has been real.

The thing I loved about Noom is I could understand it. The psychology behind it was very important to me, as I'm an emotional eater.

They were able to help me view food as fuel for my very capable body. I respect that and started to respect myself enough to look after my body better. The science they gave us satisfied my very analytical mind too.

And, overall the flow on effects towards my mental health improved too.
To be honest, I struggled with the calorie recording towards the end. But by that stage, 6 months later, I'd already lost 20kg and was stoked.

Today I'm still using a lot of what I learnt from Noom. I'm recording my 'fuel intake' and have expanded that to movement, hydration, gratitude and habits. Being mindful of what I do to look after myself is key.

Noom started a new era for me. 'No more self-abandonment'.
Happy days xx "

It Helped me Grow while Becoming Slimmer

I am delighted to introduce a very special person in my life, my husband Bogdan. Living under the same roof, we share more than just space; we share the highs and lows, meals, joys, sorrows, and the beautiful chaos that life brings. Throughout my journey of engaging in a new path to weight loss, my husband played a crucial role.

Being attentive and supportive, he observed my progress keenly for several months. Witnessing the changes and the positive impact, he not only started believing in the method but also caught the enthusiasm. His observant nature turned into active participation as he began taking mental notes of my journey.

Eventually, he became convinced that he too wanted to jump on this new life-changing journey. Today, he is here to share his story, the challenges he faced, the victories he celebrated, and the incredible results he achieved.

Without further ado, let me hand it over to him to share his inspiring journey and the remarkable transformation he underwent.

"I was 90 kgs on 13th March when I started. I was 80 kgs on 18th May when I reached my goal. I went even further down to 75 kgs by 1st August, and maintained this weight to date, almost 3 years later.

I really liked the program because it gave me one simple interface with all the advice and all the tracking tools required. From your group you learn that your challenges are not unique and also that if you stick to the program you do really well (even in comparison).

One of the things I both learned and liked is that nothing is out of reach, but you need to understand what it means to you.

I struggled with measuring and weighing everything for the first two weeks or so. I also struggled with some hunger sensation throughout the day towards the end of the first month, but that went away eventually.

It definitely helped me grow - while becoming slimmer - and understand some concepts around not only eating well, but for instance stress impact, sleeping well and exercising - and how they fit together."

Feeling in Control

I am delighted to introduce my lovely colleague, Tricia, whose untiring support and shared experiences have made our professional journey very special. Tricia and I have formed a bond that goes beyond the workplace as we rely on each other's knowledge and expertise across a spectrum of topics, ranging from children and school to travel, gardening, business, and social media – there's hardly a subject we haven't talked about.

A few years ago, during my weight loss adventure, Tricia became an integral part of my journey. She couldn't help but catch the contagious enthusiasm and positive vibes that surrounded me during that time. Inspired by the power of personal growth, she embarked on her own program and experienced a significant change in her life.

Tricia graciously agreed to share her thoughts on this experience, and her testimonial speaks volumes about the impact of embracing change and personal growth.

"When I started my weight loss journey with Noom, like many other people I had tried a lot of different weight loss programs. The difference with Noom, was I always felt in control rather than just following a program. I lost 10 kgs in 8 months which was a good pace for my body and age. I have always been very slow at losing weight.

As well as weight loss I gained knowledge about how my mind, body, stress and environment all work together for weight loss and wellbeing.

The knowledge I gained from Noom was a positive experience for me."

As emphasized earlier in this book, my purpose and goal are not to advocate for Noom as a one-size-fits-all weight loss solution. Instead, my focus was on providing you with tools that empower you to succeed and cultivate the motivation to embrace any weight loss method that aligns with your individual preferences. Recognizing the uniqueness of each individual, blindly following a program is rarely effective. The key is to invest the effort in discovering what suits you, what brings you joy, and what aligns with your desired outcomes. Get the tools provided and embark on the journey to create your own reality, tailored to your needs and aspirations.

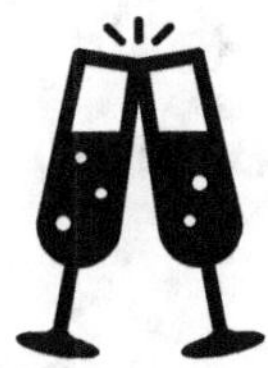

Chapter Eighteen

From Dreams to Reality: A Heartfelt Finale to Our Journey Together

As my weight loss journey unfolded, I found myself on an unexpected path of transformation that extended far beyond the magic numbers on the scale. The positive ripples of change touched every corner of my life, bringing about a cascade of improvements and newfound joys.

One of the most profound shifts occurred in my relationships. The strengthened bond with my daughter became a testament to the positive energy radiating from my newfound vitality. My husband and friends, witnessing my commitment to self-improvement, joined me in celebrating the journey towards a healthier, happier version of myself.

Embracing physical activities like gym workouts and running not only became integral to my weight loss journey but marked the inception of a fulfilling fitness adventure. The momentum from my healthier lifestyle even translated into a career shift, where I proudly assumed the role of Chief Happiness Officer at work. In my personal life, fuelled by my passion for wellbeing, I found myself exploring the realms of happiness and mindfulness, incorporating practices like daily gratitude, meditation, and the powerful tool of visualization into my routine.

Visualization became my secret weapon, a way to imagine and re-program my brain to work with me towards a slimmer, healthier, and happier version of myself. I could see myself making positive food choices, enjoying invigorating workouts, winning races, and being happy, embracing a vibrant, joyful life.

Navigating the twists and turns of this journey, I discovered the importance of patience and self-compassion. Plateaus and challenging days became part of the process, and I learned to view them as opportunities for growth. Science-backed insights reminded me that sometimes, counterintuitive actions like eating more could propel progress.

Crucially, I learned to be kind to myself on the tougher days. Understanding that a misstep in exercise or nutrition did not define my journey allowed me to bounce back with renewed determination. The wisdom of 'Noom' echoed in my mind: it wasn't about a predefined program but the tools to unlock the success already embedded in my own mind.

As I conclude this journey, I carry with me not only a lighter weight but a heart brimming with gratitude, a mind fortified by self-confidence, and a spirit fuelled by the resilience to make mindful choices for my mental and physical wellbeing. My weight loss wasn't just about shedding pounds—it was a journey of self-discovery, empowerment, and the firm belief that investing in oneself produces the most rewarding dividends. May your journey be as transformative, inspiring, and full of unexpected joys as mine has been. Here's to a healthier, happier you.

Resources

The Noom Mindset: Learn the Science, Lose the Weight
The Noom App
Dr Libby: Women's Wellness Wisdom
Accidentally Overweight: Solve Your Weight Loss Puzzle, Libby Weaver
Real Food Kitchen, Libby Weaver
Don't Lose Your Mind, Lose Your Weight, Rujuta Diwekar
Eat to live, Joel Fuhrman
Run Fast. Cook Fast. Eat Slow. Quick-Fix Recipes for Hangry Athletes: A Cookbook
The Longevity Paradox. How to Die Young at a Ripe Old Age, Steven R Gundry
The Good Life, Lessons from the World's Longest Study on Happiness, Robert Waldinger, Marc Schulz

Helpful journals and logbooks

Join me, Pink Wool, on an amazing journey towards happiness and wellbeing. As a passionate advocate, I like exploring the realm of self-development, fitness and mindfulness, sharing my knowledge through an array of books, including gratitude journals, logbooks, planners, and even coloring books. Beyond personal growth, my mission extends to fostering a healthier and more compassionate society, promoting habits that cultivate wellbeing, joy, gratitude, and mindfulness. By following me, you become part of a community dedicated to creating a fulfilling life through simple, actionable steps. Explore my Amazon profile for a collection of books tailored for those seeking personal growth, productivity, and increased happiness. Let's embark on this adventure together and make positive changes, one habit at a time. Follow me now and be part of the movement for personal growth and wellbeing!

https://www.amazon.com/author/pinkwool

THANK YOU!

Thank you for joining me on this journey. If you've enjoyed this book, I invite you to check out my other journals, notebooks and coloring books on my Amazon Author Page. Your support means the world to me and I can't wait to share more adventures with you. Happy exploring!

Go to: https://www.amazon.com/author/pinkwool

Or scan this QR Code:

Also if you liked this book, please consider leaving a review. It only takes a few seconds and helps my small business in a huge way! Simply scan this QR Code: